I0782626

# LOSING WEIGHT

## THE SAFE & SMART PATH

ISBN-13: 978-1986823562

ISBN-10: 1986823563

information: www.thefreewindows.com

Steven Adams

# Losing Weight

## The Safe & Smart path

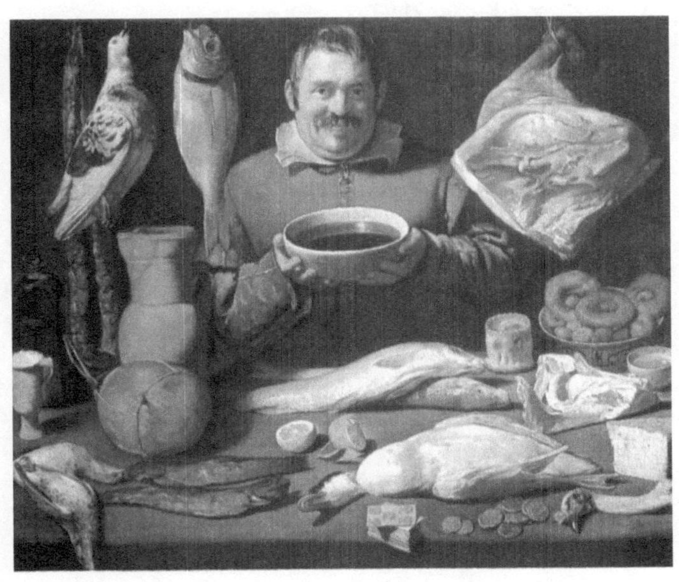

# Contents

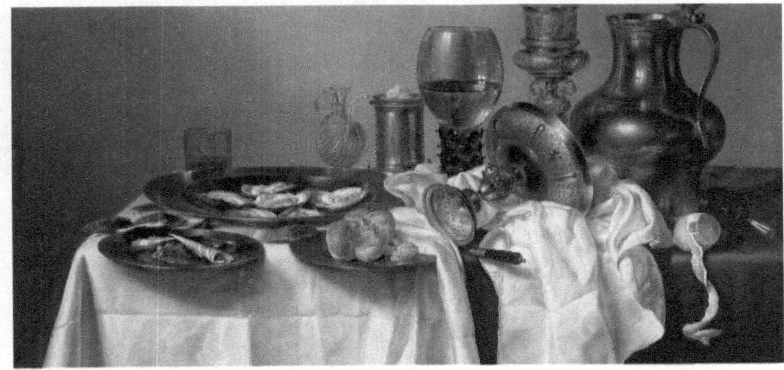

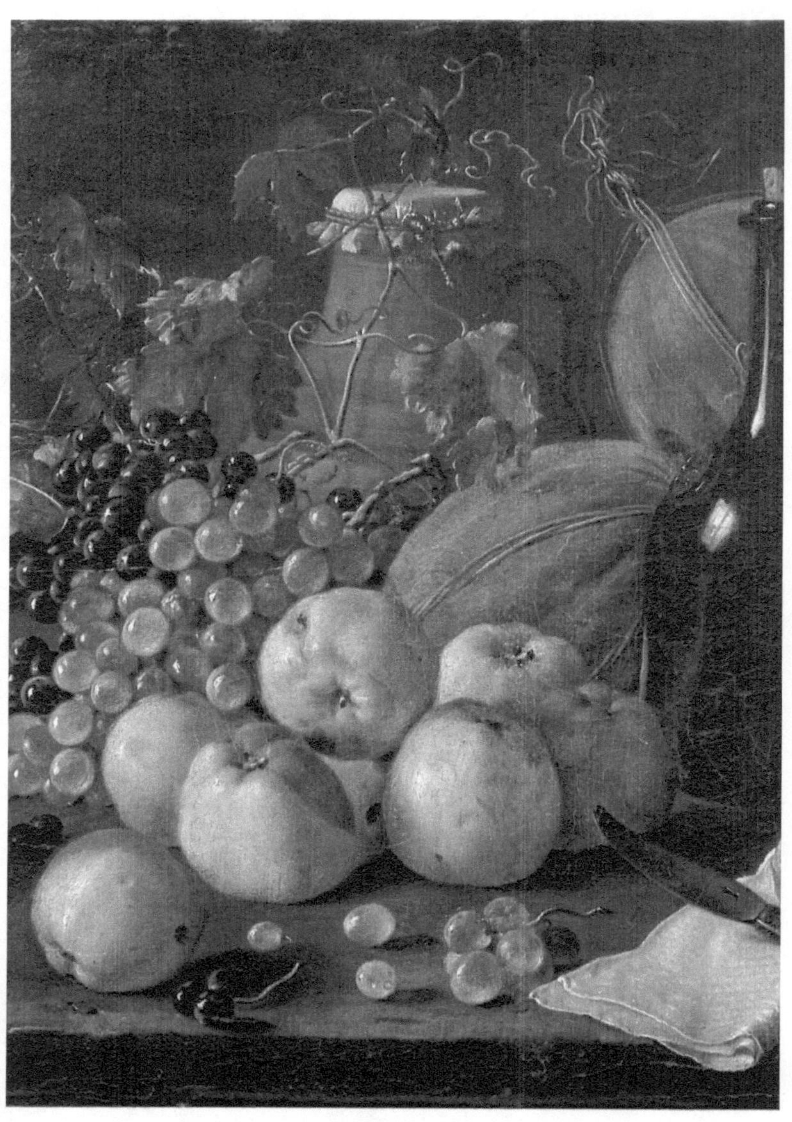

*I absolutely hate being fat!* I feel disfigured, guilty, entrapped, disappointed... I fear for my health and I suffer already. When I am with fat people who eat a lot, is like seeing myself — irresponsible, weak, suffering, irrational... I don't know if I should be sorry or angry.

My normal weight is about 150 lb. (68 kg) and I managed to become 210 (95 kg)! You do not get there in a week, but strange as it may seem, you *can* ignore the problem until people start telling you, or your health collapses! At least this is what happened with me.

I didn't realize how I became fat! Obviously sometime I started buying new clothes, but I don't remember when, I was not seriously alarmed, I didn't have a real awareness of my situation, I had not devoted any time at all to think about this problem, to realize the causes and free myself!

Even if you lose weight, it's not impossible to gain it back, now being aware, yet *pathetically* unable to respond... Until sometime your health or your shape or your friends force you to do something.

In this book I share my experience of what worked for me, what I did trying to lose weight, reading and thinking about dishes, habits, calories, diets, health, and anything relevant, for a long time.

I ate and still eat *whatever* I like —even pizza and sweets!— and I don't let myself feel hungry. But I am now aware all the time of the real problem and of the real enemy in this weight–loss battle.

---

*Fat is only a consequence of the defeat, not the enemy.*

---

*Your goal should never be only to lose weight,* but to get rid of the problem that is behind weight gain.

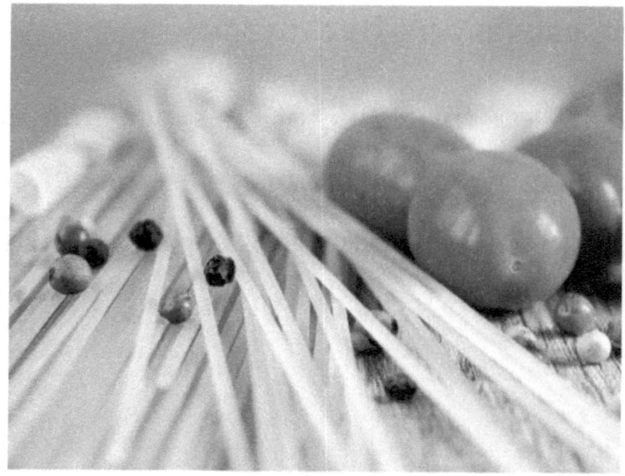

# The war is against gluttony and dullness

In this book I take for granted that you checked thoroughly and you are sure you don't suffer from a biological disease making you gain weight. If your problem is *not* that you eat too much without reason, you don't need this book.

I suffer from gluttony. When I realized the problem, I began to form also a clear understanding of what I had to do, even to avoid gaining back the weight I would hopefully lose.

Gluttony is the urge to satisfy palate and belly, an illness that has been considered even a deadly sin: gluttony is to surrender oneself to the pleasure of taste, when you are always ready to think of food, eager to eat what you like and to fill yourself completely...

*"The majority are glutted like beasts"*, says the Greek philosopher Heraclitus, showing that we refer to a reality that surpasses a simple fitness is-

sue: *gluttony can subordinate our mind*, and this devotion to a lower object underestimates us, is a betrayal of our better self.

---

*The power of gluttony is great, because its cause is internal and not easily realized.*

---

Self-enslavement, this most important consequence of gluttony is described vividly in a story about the ancient philosopher D i o g e n e s.

One day, Diogenes ate a dish of lentils while sitting on the threshold of a random house. In ancient Greece, if someone ate lentils for a meal, a very cheap and common food, it meant that he was in a state of destitution. An emissary from the prince's entourage passing by said: *"Ah! Diogenes, if only you tried not to be so contumacious towards our prince, but more of a flatterer, you would not be forced to eat lentils all the time."* Diogenes looked up into the eyes of his rich interlocutor, and responded: *"Oh, my poor brother! If only you learnt to eat a few lentils, you would not be forced to obey and flatter the prince all the time."*

This story reminded me of movies like The Firm, where a company spoils its lawyers, offering a life of pleasure for them and their families. Their love for luxury made them ready to succumb to crime in order to support what became for them an irresistible addiction. Tom Cruise resisted this temptation, and you can do the same.

Does this mean we should give up all pleasure and be satisfied with what we like less? On the contrary!

Especially if seen as a psychological problem, *fighting gluttony is about gaining freedom*: food or *lack of it* should not determine our will. We cannot let a dependence on unpleasant food become necessary for controlling our appetite.

The problem in gluttony is not with pleasure, but with *addiction*. You can have pleasure and be ready to give it up when you need to, or you can sacrifice for pleasure your health, your freedom, your dignity...

Ancient Greeks emphasize m e a s u r e, and this became a key concept in my fat and gluttony problem. I knew that, especially if I wanted my freedom back, I should find a way to combine pleasure with measure — eat whatever I like, and stop before I was *glutted like beasts...*

---

*One thing is to understand that you need to eat less; it is different, stronger and more important, to do it as a way to be free.*

---

Gluttony is not another name for the pleasure of taste and fulfilment; it is the eagerness to obtain this pleasure and the readiness to sacrifice for it things more significant, such as your health.

As you can see, gluttony resembles smoke addiction, both habits enslave but there is also a great difference.

*Smoking offers an illusory pleasure,* actually being nothing more than complying with the addiction to a harmful drug; food offers a real pleasure and is even useful. Food with a lot of calories, such as nuts or dark chocolate, contribute to a healthy life, requiring only a little caution. Alcohol itself is beneficial if consumed moderately.

Being a source of health and of real pleasure, food can become steadily alluring even more than smoke. Awareness of this 'mechanism' helps to develop a stronger sense of what it takes to eat less, lose weight and be free.

*I just quit and forgot about smoking once and for all, but how can I fight eating, when each and every day I taste and enjoy and my desire grows?*

Realizing this I concluded that most of all I should not allow myself to feel hungry or to stop enjoying food.

Thus I arrived to the problem of negativity.

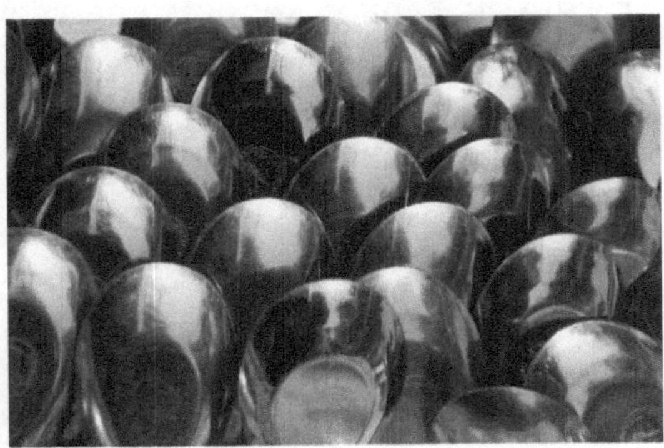

# Negativity is a great enemy

Putting some effort to achieve a goal has a positive meaning: I do something that leads to a result. I take an aspirin to stop my headache, I study to learn, I put on this coat to fight cold... A critical problem with weight loss is that *you need to do nothing, you need to n o t eat!*

I don't doubt, if there was a real, working and safe p i l l for losing weight, fat people would be fewer and the fight against obesity *a lot* easier.

As was said, the problem becomes greater by the fact that eating is a real pleasure, food a real and necessary good. Thus, on one side you have *a b s t i - n e n c e*, a negative force, and on the other you have eating, a positive activity, permanent and necessary.

Unfair fight! It cannot support the feeling that you do something, that you act! Note that in this regard too weight loss resembles the struggle to quit smoking.

As all passionate smokers know, their ideal condition would be that of *chain smoking*. A lot of them do precisely this, ruining their health along with their self-esteem, but those who are a little prudent try to let some time pass before they satisfy their addiction.

However — and this is the most important here to note — the prudent time of abstinence, their useful and healthy time, is regarded by smokers mainly as wasted, empty and vain, tragically opposed to the 'positive' time of smoking, this one being essentially identified as a time of pleasure and satisfaction!

Dealing with this problem when I was smoking, dramatically more when I decided to quit smoking, I tried to realize and appreciate the necessary abstinence as full of immediate positive consequences, a condition that revealed something so subtle, you couldn't tell it was there before: I tried to start enjoying the simple, beneficial and always present a i r instead of smoke.

In quitting smoking one gains an experience of health improvement even in a couple of days, but in weight loss things are not easy, especially in the beginning, when all benefits, no matter how certainly known, remain just information about an *expected* condition, a reality of a happy *future*, not only in the appearance of one's body, but also in health.

Is there any way out of this difficulty? Is there anything we can immediately enjoy as we suppress our appetite, a 'hidden' reality that could emerge now for us in the place of taste, offering some alternative satisfaction and comfort?

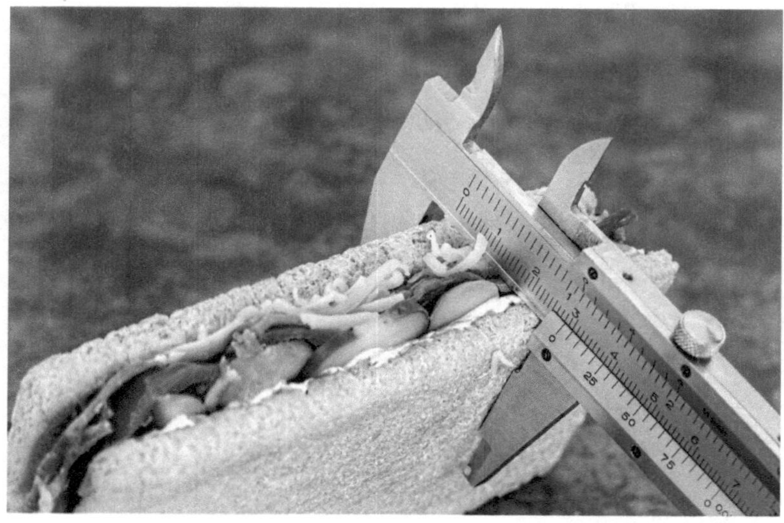

# Weight loss as a positive experience

As anyone starting this fight, I tried to concentrate on weight loss *as health gain and shape gain*, but I soon realized I needed more than that, something I could sense right now instead of relying on hope only.

Thus I appreciated even more what I call *weight loss allies*.

I began to understand them also as providers of a justified impression that you actually do something besides not eating.

For instance, exercise is not only a great way to burn extra calories, it gives a strength that you can feel immediately, and increasingly in the course of time, letting you experience a self that is less fat and more able, even before you are indeed less fat and more able!

The rest of the allies I select here as being most useful, won't give you perhaps a sense of a better self, but they will support you in your need to feel that you do something, that you act, instead of just not eating and waiting for the miracle to happen.

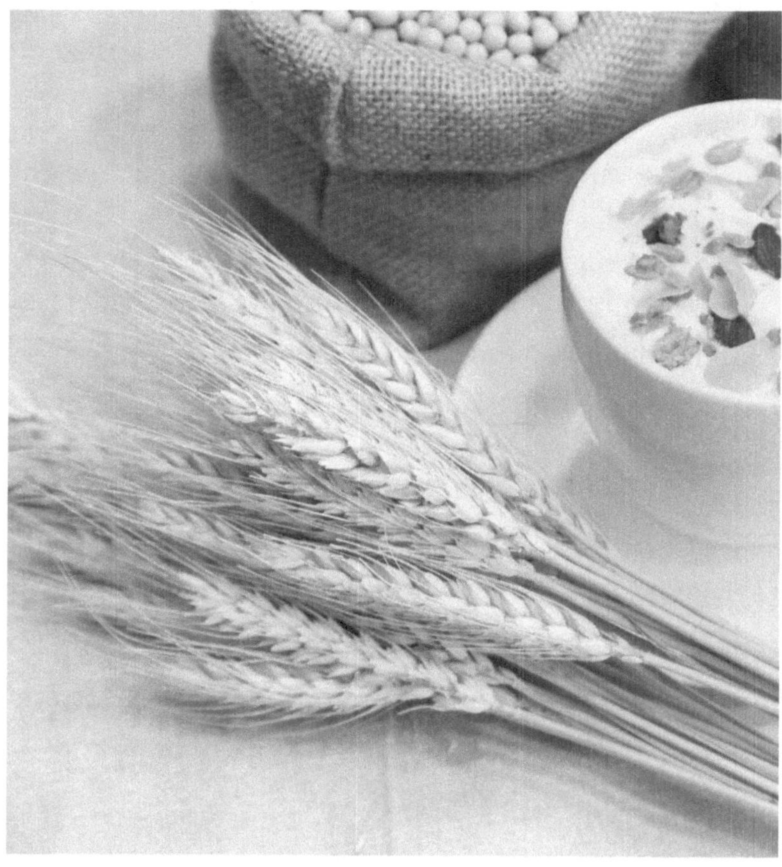

# Weight loss allies

'Allies' prevent excessive eating, some of them even allow a sense of victory in advance, or at least, if you neglect your purpose, a foretaste of your failure that becomes a warning.

## *The scale*

A quality scale, able to detect differences of about 0.2 lb. (about 100 g), is necessary and is a great ally.

In a day you can gain or lose about 1 lb. (453 g) the most; it helps to monitor your progress daily, be-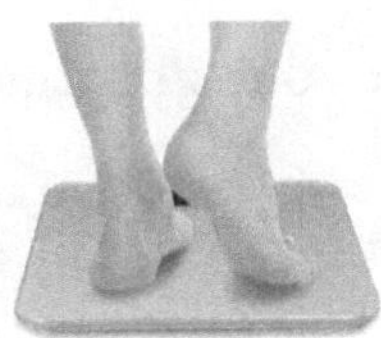cause you get in your everyday life something 'tangible', a real sense of where you are, what you achieve or how much you fail.

Waiting for the end of a whole week to learn where you are, your progress becomes vague, you feel like you walk in a mist, without a sense of satisfaction when your scale testifies that your efforts in the previous day were fruitful and brought you closer to your goal.

This should be clear from the start: *weight loss needs time*, even more if you won't follow an austere diet, which you shouldn't do anyway.

---

*Your most immediate purpose and satisfaction, should be to lose about 0.33 lb. (approx. 150 g) daily.*

---

First thing I understood as I guess everyone with a weight problem: it's easy to gain weight until you find yourself fat, but difficult to lose even a little each day until you return to your normal condition.

In this regard it helps to know that *your greatest obstacle is your very progress!*

When I started losing weight I became self–confident in a disastrous way, I developed a tendency to abandon my healthy habits, as if getting thinner were an automatic process, something that would keep going on without my participation!

Of course I started to become fat again and I realized that I needed to hold myself tight to this rational measure which proved able to help me lose weight.

The real paradox is that the cycle of *success > pseudo–confidence > relaxation > failure > remorse* can be repeated a lot of times! It seems that realizing it is indeed possible for you to succeed in this effort, you provide yourself a motive to *postpone* your discipline and surrender to gluttony! Since you *are* able, you don't have anything to fear! Until you find yourself so fat, that losing weight seems again impossible, in which case, especially after several failures, you might not even return to your healthy decisions, abandoning hope completely.

Understanding this mechanism of *relaxation and failure* is essential, if one wants to avoid unnecessary delays or even disappointment.

Note also that it's greater and even more valuable not only to lose weight but to gain dietary habits that will let you *keep* your normal weight in the future.

## The mirror

In a mirror you realize better your shape, comparing it with how you should or used to be.

It is natural to care for that. How we look is not a weaker motive than health for losing weight, because it influences our personal and professional relationships.

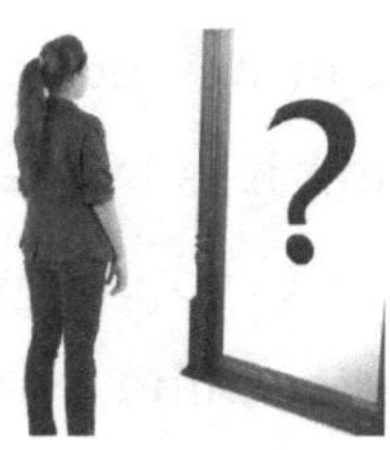

An identification with one's own image is a cause of problems, not only because we are more than our appearance, but because we change, wanting it or not and causing it or not, *we age* even remaining thin. However, there is no need to make things worse by adding fat to whatever time brings!

# Sleep

Sleep is such a great ally! We tend to feel hungry at night, even after a full evening meal, because by the end of the day we are tired. This is crucial. A lot of people report that they fail to control their appetite at night! It's not real hunger but lack of a strength that comes with sleep.

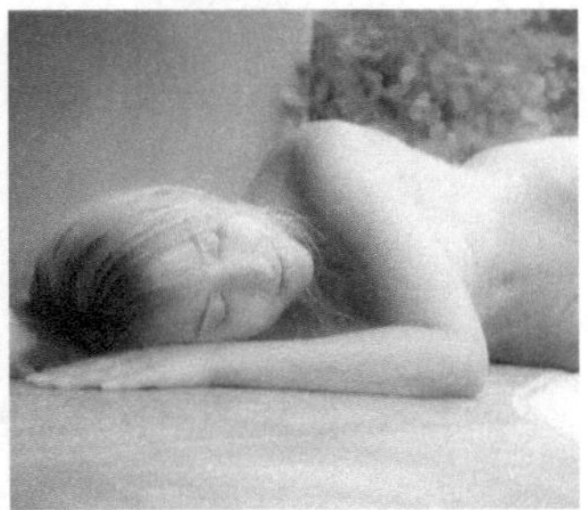

*Avoid eating at night, fool your supposed hunger with a handful of nuts until you go to sleep and give yourself what it really needs.*

An adult should sleep about 8 hours a day, but make sure you enjoy q u a l i t y sleep hours, in a dark, comfortable and silent room.

Note that if you suffer from sleepiness during the day or feel tired, although you slept enough, you need to consult your physician.

## Water

Water is an important ally, even more than sleep. Sometimes you cannot sleep as much as you need, but water you can drink whenever. Water is not 'charged' with calories, you may drink as much as you like, and more!

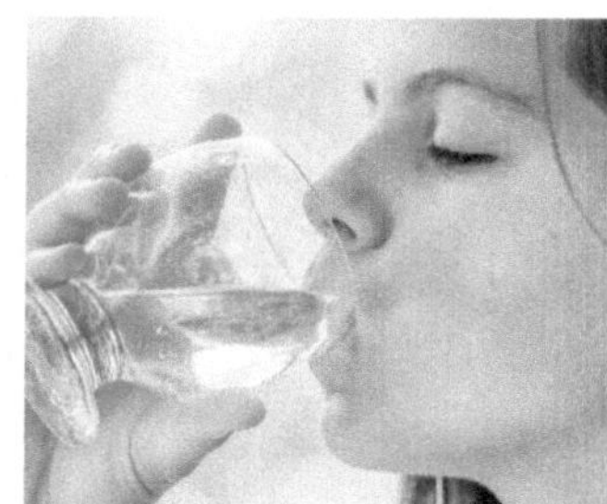

There is a specific use of water that saved me from a lot of trouble. My biggest problem with weight loss was those pangs, especially at night or late in the evening. But even during the day pangs exist and should be avoided.

*Never eat unless you are certain your hunger is real.*

When a hunger pang appears, drink a glass of water and let 10 minutes pass. If you are still hungry, eat as much as it takes *to reduce and postpone your appetite,* not to feel satiated. When you feel hungry you may like (and be able) to eat, for instance, 3 toasts with cheese. If you eat just one and wait for 10 minutes, your appetite will be lost and you will have avoided more than 500 calories.

Thus I eat a lot of times, always small quantities, allowing myself to eat anything, quality food — with a few exceptions.

Even when we order a pizza, I stop at the second piece, but usually I make myself a personal pizza in a way that minimizes its calories and increases its quality. More on this later, at my weekly schedule.

It's more important than anything, taking into account that gluttony is the great enemy, to have in mind the fleeting nature of the pleasure of eating.

---

*Enjoy your favorite food, but do not try to perpetuate this joy by eating more and more...*

---

*We don't need much of anything*, Peter Gabriel sings wisely. Your favorite taste lasts only while you eat and a couple of minutes more, but the fat you store in your body is there to stay, until, perhaps, you find the strength to control your habits and get rid of it.

## Coffee

Coffee postpones the feeling of hunger. Just coffee — without cream or anything full of calories! You may use some milk and sug- 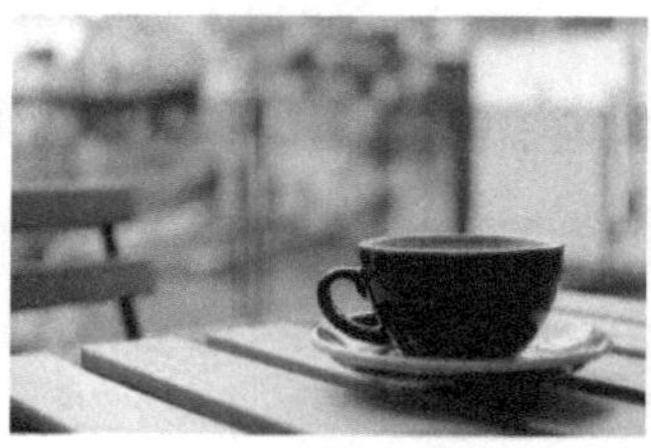 ar or honey, but check what you add — do not transform one of your greatest allies into a primary source of fat!

## Exercise

Doctors agree, exercise improves our health so much, that overcomes our being a *little* overweight. If we had to choose between losing a few pounds and devoting some time to exercise, we should always choose the second. But of course it's easy to have them both.

---

*Exercise improved my health more than I ever expected! I was afraid to run, even to walk, because I had become fragile.*

---

Especially my knees and legs were so infirm, I could not trust them. If I had a chance to walk a bit faster for just a couple of meters, I n e v e r did it, preferring to wait for the proper traffic lights!

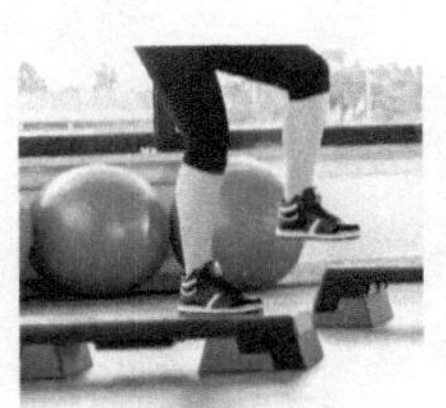

Now I cross the street run-ning, even if I have only a *risky* chance! But now I do some exercise every day, and I am also in my normal weight.

I'm not an athletic type, otherwise I wouldn't have become fat, I guess. By *exercising* I don't mean (and I didn't need) anything exhaustive or excessive!

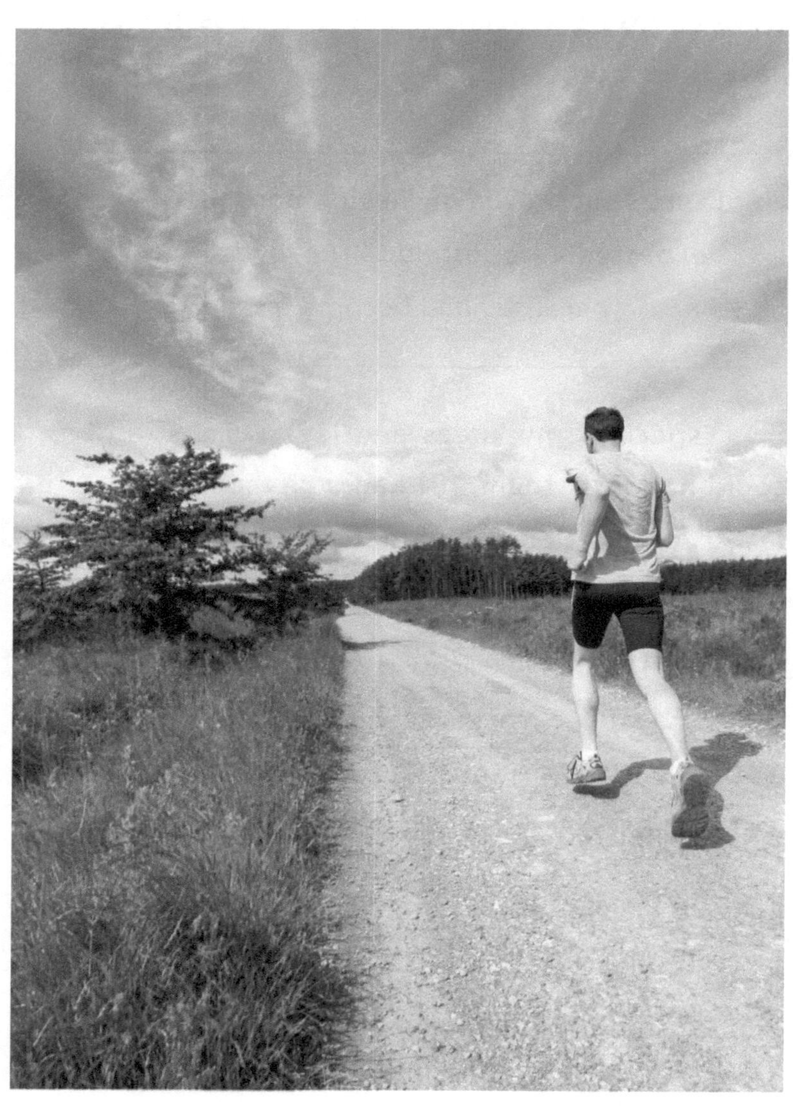

*Exercise bores me*, I must confess, and I never followed a method in a gym or at home. What I did was to just stop watching my favorite movies sitting in the sofa!

I combine movie time with exercise, using a stepper. You could use a bike, a treadmill or anything similar. Once in a while I stop 'walking' and continue with weights (still watching my movie). I started from a 3 kg unit in the first weeks. When that became easy, I went to 5 and now I am and most probably I will remain to 7 kg (about 15 lb.).

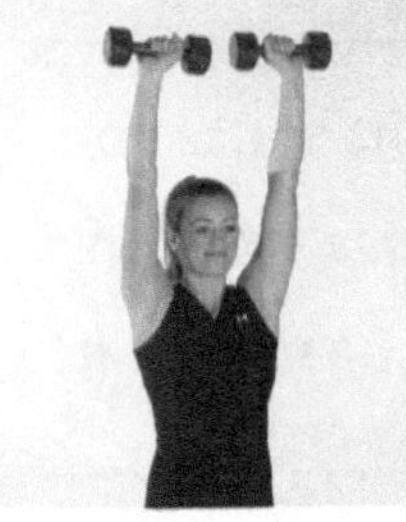

If you enjoy a better physical condition you can use two units. I preferred just one to prolong my exercise by changing hand. Using two units you find both hands simultaneously tired, which leaves you waiting until you are able to go on.

Note that *light lifting*, such as vinyl dumbbells, is *aerobic* exercise; it allows and needs many repetitions or 'sets', as they are called, that make you breath more intensely for more time. Don't confuse this type of exercise with heavy lifting, where athletes are trained to handle the heaviest possible weight just once.

Any exercise is great, even a simple walk outside. If you feel bored, just use those earphones to listen to your favorite music.

As you lose weight, day by day, exercise helps not only by burning calories and giving strength but also because it lets you feel intensely your body getting better.

*Exercise creates conditions that contribute to your confidence. Just make sure to use this confidence to fulfil your goal and not to postpone it!*

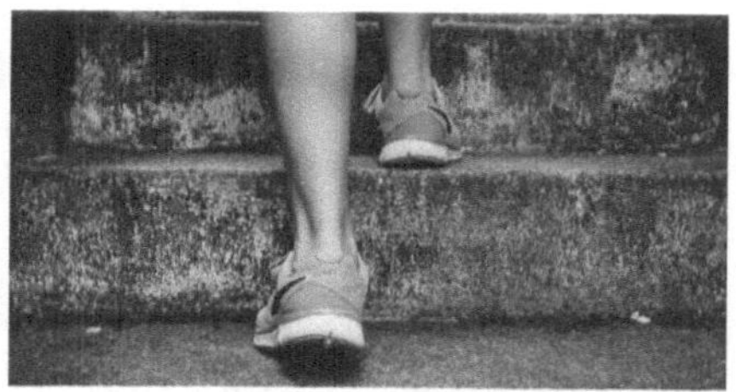

Here is a table with the amount of calories you can burn in some activities.

# Calories burned with exercise

Male and female, in various ages and frames, burn different amounts of calories. This table (based on a middle condition) can be used only as an indicative approximation.

| 1 hour of exercise ||| | Calories |
| --- | --- |
| Hiking | 400 |
| Gardening / yard work | 330 |
| Bicycling (< 10 mph) | 290 |
| Walking (3.5 mph) | 300 |
| Light weight training | 220 |
| Stretching | 180 |
| Elliptical trainer, moderate effort | 360 |
| Stair Step | 420 |

## Vigorous activities

| | Calories |
| --- | --- |
| Jogging (4.5 mph) | 600 |
| Bicycling (> 10 mph) | 590 |
| Swimming (slow) | 510 |
| Tennis | 520 |
| Aerobics | 480 |
| Walking (5 mph) | 460 |
| Heavy yard work | 440 |
| Vigorous weight lifting | 440 |

# Health

Obesity means a greater risk of finding yourself with diabetes, high blood pressure, heart strokes, cancer, kidney impairment, sleep apnea...

Childhood obesity is the reason why even kids and teens are so much affected by diabetes.

It was common knowledge once, that being a little overweight adds life years! It's not a paradox, it's just not true.

Actually normal weight helps you to prevent cardiovascular disease and the trouble that comes with it. Not to mention diseases like cancer.

However, I prefer personally to think less about those serious diseases, because anyway obesity becomes a real problem: it would not let me even *walk* normally!

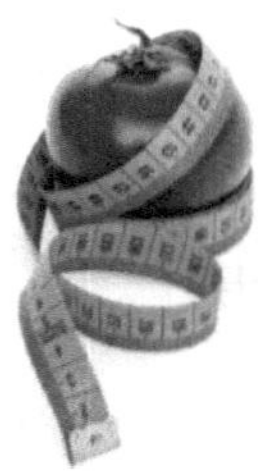

# Your ideal weight

Normal or 'ideal' weight differs according to age, gender, and the type or 'frame' of your body.

A quick method to realize if you are fat and how much, is to determine your body mass index, or BMI as is known. It's described by the formula

$$Weight / Height^2$$

where weight is expressed in kilograms and height in meters. All you need is just a simple calculator.

First find the square of your height. For instance, if you are 1.6 meters tall, multiply 1.6 by itself. This gives you 2.56.

Then divide your weight by 2.56. For instance, if you are 70 kg heavy, dividing 70 by 2.56 gives you 27.3, which is your BMI.

What is the meaning of this number?

Underweight = less than 18.5

Normal weight = 18.5–24.9

Overweight = 25–29.9

Obesity = 30 or greater

Therefore, having a BMI of 27.3 you are overweight, but not obese. Just lose some pounds, until your BMI is less than 25, but no need to rush.

Regardless of the calculation above, in the following charts you can find approximately your ideal weight range according to your *sex, height* and *frame.*

Men

| | Height | | | Weight | | | | | Small Frame | | | | | Medium Frame | | | | | Large Frame | | |
|---|---|---|---|---|---|---|---|---|---|---|---|---|---|---|---|---|---|---|---|---|
| (ft) | (in) | (cm) | (lbs) | - | (lbs) | (kg) | - | (kg) | (lbs) | - | (lbs) | (kg) | - | (kg) | (lbs) | - | (lbs) | (kg) | - | (kg) |
| 4 | 10 | 147 | 102 | - | 111 | 46 | - | 50 | 109 | - | 121 | 49 | - | 55 | 118 | - | 131 | 54 | - | 59 |
| 4 | 11 | 150 | 103 | - | 113 | 47 | - | 51 | 111 | - | 123 | 50 | - | 56 | 120 | - | 134 | 54 | - | 61 |
| 5 | 0 | 153 | 104 | - | 115 | 47 | - | 52 | 113 | - | 126 | 51 | - | 57 | 122 | - | 137 | 55 | - | 62 |
| 5 | 1 | 155 | 106 | - | 118 | 48 | - | 54 | 115 | - | 129 | 52 | - | 59 | 125 | - | 140 | 57 | - | 64 |
| 5 | 2 | 158 | 108 | - | 121 | 49 | - | 55 | 118 | - | 132 | 54 | - | 60 | 128 | - | 143 | 58 | - | 65 |
| 5 | 3 | 160 | 111 | - | 124 | 50 | - | 56 | 121 | - | 135 | 55 | - | 61 | 131 | - | 147 | 59 | - | 67 |
| 5 | 4 | 163 | 114 | - | 127 | 52 | - | 58 | 124 | - | 138 | 56 | - | 63 | 134 | - | 151 | 61 | - | 68 |
| 5 | 5 | 165 | 117 | - | 130 | 53 | - | 59 | 127 | - | 141 | 58 | - | 64 | 137 | - | 155 | 62 | - | 70 |
| 5 | 6 | 168 | 120 | - | 133 | 54 | - | 60 | 130 | - | 144 | 59 | - | 65 | 140 | - | 159 | 64 | - | 72 |
| 5 | 7 | 170 | 123 | - | 136 | 56 | - | 62 | 133 | - | 147 | 60 | - | 67 | 143 | - | 163 | 65 | - | 74 |
| 5 | 8 | 173 | 126 | - | 139 | 57 | - | 63 | 136 | - | 150 | 62 | - | 68 | 146 | - | 167 | 66 | - | 76 |
| 5 | 9 | 175 | 129 | - | 142 | 59 | - | 64 | 139 | - | 153 | 63 | - | 69 | 149 | - | 170 | 68 | - | 77 |
| 5 | 10 | 178 | 132 | - | 145 | 60 | - | 66 | 142 | - | 156 | 64 | - | 71 | 152 | - | 173 | 69 | - | 78 |
| 5 | 11 | 180 | 135 | - | 148 | 61 | - | 67 | 145 | - | 159 | 66 | - | 72 | 155 | - | 176 | 70 | - | 80 |
| 6 | 0 | 183 | 138 | - | 151 | 63 | - | 68 | 148 | - | 162 | 67 | - | 73 | 158 | - | 179 | 72 | - | 81 |

## Women

| Height | | | Weight | | | | | | | | | | | | | | |
| --- | --- | --- | --- | --- | --- | --- | --- | --- | --- | --- | --- | --- | --- | --- | --- | --- | --- |
| | | | Small Frame | | | | | | Medium Frame | | | | | | Large Frame | | |
| (ft) | (in) | (cm) | (lbs) | | (lbs) | (kg) | | (kg) | (lbs) | | (lbs) | (kg) | | (kg) | (lbs) | | (lbs) | (kg) | | (kg) |
| 5 | 2 | 158 | 128 | - | 134 | 58 | - | 61 | 131 | - | 141 | 59 | - | 64 | 138 | - | 150 | 63 | - | 68 |
| 5 | 3 | 160 | 130 | - | 136 | 59 | - | 62 | 133 | - | 143 | 60 | - | 65 | 140 | - | 153 | 64 | - | 69 |
| 5 | 4 | 163 | 132 | - | 138 | 60 | - | 63 | 135 | - | 145 | 61 | - | 66 | 142 | - | 156 | 64 | - | 71 |
| 5 | 5 | 165 | 134 | - | 140 | 61 | - | 64 | 137 | - | 148 | 62 | - | 67 | 144 | - | 160 | 65 | - | 73 |
| 5 | 6 | 168 | 136 | - | 142 | 62 | - | 64 | 139 | - | 151 | 63 | - | 68 | 146 | - | 164 | 66 | - | 74 |
| 5 | 7 | 170 | 138 | - | 145 | 63 | - | 66 | 142 | - | 154 | 64 | - | 70 | 149 | - | 168 | 68 | - | 76 |
| 5 | 8 | 173 | 140 | - | 148 | 64 | - | 67 | 145 | - | 157 | 66 | - | 71 | 152 | - | 172 | 69 | - | 78 |
| 5 | 9 | 175 | 142 | - | 151 | 64 | - | 68 | 148 | - | 160 | 67 | - | 73 | 155 | - | 176 | 70 | - | 80 |
| 5 | 10 | 178 | 144 | - | 154 | 65 | - | 70 | 151 | - | 163 | 68 | - | 74 | 158 | - | 180 | 72 | - | 82 |
| 5 | 11 | 180 | 146 | - | 157 | 66 | - | 71 | 154 | - | 166 | 70 | - | 75 | 161 | - | 184 | 73 | - | 83 |
| 6 | 0 | 183 | 149 | - | 160 | 68 | - | 73 | 157 | - | 170 | 71 | - | 77 | 164 | - | 188 | 74 | - | 85 |
| 6 | 1 | 186 | 152 | - | 164 | 69 | - | 74 | 160 | - | 174 | 73 | - | 79 | 168 | - | 192 | 76 | - | 87 |
| 6 | 2 | 188 | 155 | - | 168 | 70 | - | 76 | 164 | - | 178 | 74 | - | 81 | 172 | - | 197 | 78 | - | 89 |
| 6 | 3 | 191 | 158 | - | 172 | 72 | - | 78 | 167 | - | 182 | 76 | - | 83 | 176 | - | 202 | 80 | - | 92 |
| 6 | 4 | 193 | 162 | - | 176 | 73 | - | 80 | 171 | - | 187 | 78 | - | 85 | 181 | - | 207 | 82 | - | 94 |

*

There is also a general rule that may be for you more convenient than these charts. Do not let yourself become heavier than what your *height-to-waist* ratio permits: *keep your waist circumference to less than half your height.* This is valid for men and women alike. For instance, if you are 152 cm (60 in) tall, your waist should be less than 76 cm (30 in).

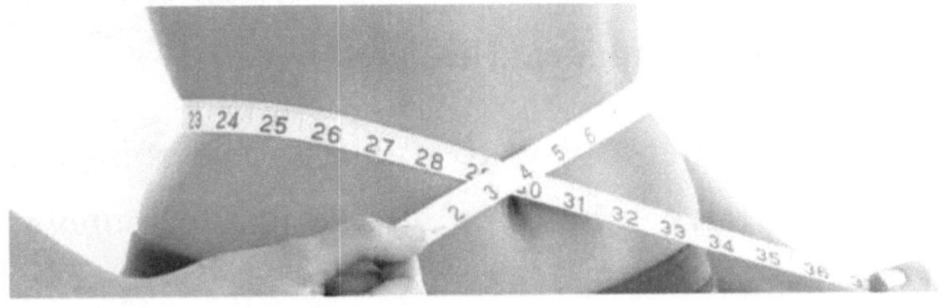

# Stop thinking of food!

If you are in love you don't think of food so much; in fact, if your occupation, or just reading a book, watching a movie — whatever you may do — fascinates you, it takes your mind away from food!

Food can never become fascinating, because it satisfies mainly taste, and temporarily.

This is bad news! If we are so absorbed by something so unable to fascinate and so able to harm, perhaps we suffer an emptiness in our life.

But this is also good news, because we now are aware of a real problem and have a chance to recognize in gluttony something more than temptations of a pleasure.

Eating can be nothing more or less than an easy way or final resort for us to remain somehow attached to the very fact that we are alive.

The very best way to reduce our appetite, would be to have something else to like *incomparably* more than food.

The same is true for smoke: it becomes extremely difficult to find the strength to quit, if you are unable to enjoy clean air, or if you live your life as if it wasn't worth living.

## Be creative!

Whatever fascinates you helps to forget about eating, and creativity *can* be fascinating!

*To be creative you need first to work from your own.*

Regardless of what you are obliged to do following the rules or needs of your profession, directions of your superiors, etc., even if your creativity is always connected with your professional life, you need to love what you do and have a passion to do more and better.

If you don't like your occupation, at least try in your free hours to let yourself be filled with thoughts and activities able to stimulate your attention and absorb you enough to forget about food.

Do you like music? *That's not enough, you need* to be excited! Listen to music you really love, if you are to use it also as a distraction from eating.

Go for a walk to let the openness comfort you! Choose books that excite you, watch movies that won't let you think about anything else.

The more interesting and exciting your life is, the less you will be thinking of food, and your gluttony will be defeated easily, without even trying!

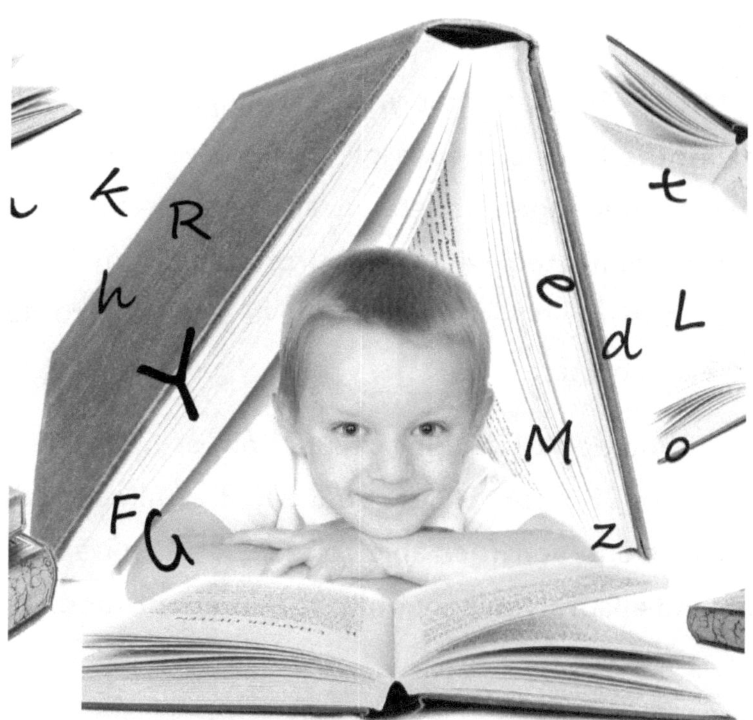

# Patience

Losing weight takes time. Two kinds of patience are necessary,

1) To accept fully that you won't reach in a few days magically your ideal weight, and

2) Not to feel satisfied after losing a few pounds, letting yourself ignore your schedule, already eating more, as if your goal had been accomplished!

The first difficulty, that the 'Day of the Ideal Weight' can be as far away as a lot of months, is not the greatest. Of course I wanted to become thin instantly, but I didn't need a lot of time to realize the hard truth.

The second problem is tougher; when I started losing weight I became so confident, so sure I can indeed achieve my goal, that I even invited back the old habits, eating more than I needed! The result was of course that I stalled for a long time, even started gaining weight.

To lose weight without the slightest risk for your health, *you need to eat everything* —quality food but everything—, *you need to eat enough* —starving isn't allowed—, and *you need time*, to lose weight slowly.

Returning to overeating or eating a lot of sweets, pies, etc., you make this already slow process even lengthier, preparing disappointment, so that you risk not only to need more time to reach your normal weight, but also to stop your efforts and become even fatter!

*Patience and perseverance* are necessary, to keep your healthy habits as long as it takes in order to reach your normal weight, and then relax them only to a degree that would let you maintain this weight.

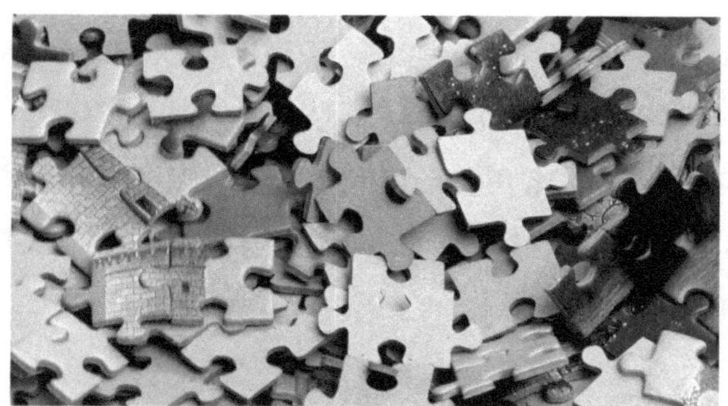

# High quality food is a first priority

Knowing that if I wanted to lose weight calories should be minimized, I realized also that most of all I had to avoid useless and even life–threatening calories, what we usually call *junk food.*

Of course high quality food can also have a lot of calories. Dark chocolate is a great example, or olive oil, or products based on sesame — tahini, halva, etc. This sort of *heavy–and–healthy* food should not be avoided, only consumed with moderation.

In the final section of this book I'm giving recipes that I used, most of them traditional in the Mediterranean cuisine, all modified by me to reduce calories and increase even more their quality, along with a weekly schedule that I followed to enjoy healthy nutritious food without undermining my objective to lose weight.

Since I managed to return to my normal weight without starving, without even excluding high–

calorie foods that I like, I'm sharing with you what I learned, knowing that it will help you as it did with me. Provided, of course, that you are really determined to lose weight.

Note that eating high quality food contains a particular psychological dimension you don't want to ignore: *it makes you feel responsible for your health, and successful in protecting it.*

By eating junk food you support the opposite inclination, an urge that most people have, to neglect your health and the overall quality of your life.

Food quality regards ingredients and safety, food that has been produced in a clean environment and is sanitized. Assuming you know where you shop from, always checking also the labels that describe product ingredients, let's recall some of your best choices.

Eat whatever vegetables and fruits you like, the more the better — in quantity and variety.

Eat any fish you like, making sure it comes from clean waters, organic farming, etc.

Prefer turkey and chicken (skinless), but you have also from time to time the liberty to enjoy red meat without fat.

Do not avoid extra virgin olive oil, a most healthy food, just don't use large quantities, because it has a lot of calories.

Nuts too are good, but they are high in calories. A handful is enough and you should not avoid it. Do not eat nuts mixed with sugar.

Eat whole wheat bread and pasta: never eat white bread or anything made with white flour!

Avoid sugar.

Don't be afraid of eggs.

It's not a crime to include small quantities of low-fat cheese in your weekly routine.

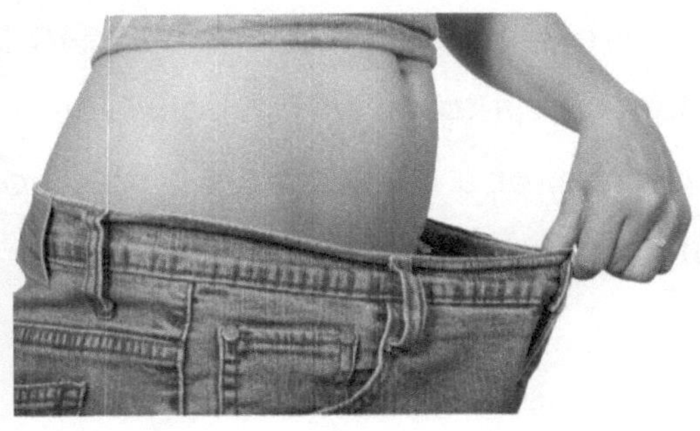

# My weekly schedule

My weekly schedule combines these elements:

1) Low fat, as possible,

2) Eating everything, but

3) Eating healthy — even with some exceptions, and

4) Always eating small quantities, mainly to lose my appetite, satisfying hunger without overeating,

5) Eating only when I am really hungry (but not starving), without keeping meticulously meal times,

6) Having no breakfast if I don't feel hungry, in which case I drink just a cup of coffee with a little honey instead of sugar. If I have breakfast, or later, near noon, whenever I start feeling hungry, I eat some oats with fresh milk, without sugar, or a couple of fried eggs, or a toast with whole wheat bread and low-fat cheese, or a tuna salad with lettuce and a tablespoon of olive-oil, etc.

7) Having no meals after 7 pm, except for a handful of nuts, a fruit, a yoghurt, and the like.

8) Eating just one 'heavy' meal a day, near 6 o'clock, and several smaller meals like breakfast, *if and when* I am hungry, mainly to lose my appetite, never to be *glutted like beasts...*

## *Monday & Thursday*

These are the days of *legumes* (aka pulses). I rotate various kinds of beans —white, broad, blackeye, green, lima—, and also peas, split peas, chickpeas, lentils... and I'm open to trying more! I just don't use two or more together, because their taste becomes then indifferent, and it's a shame, because each of them alone is delicious.

Legumes are common in the so called "Mediterranean" diet. It's a low-fat food, rich in protein, fiber, and antioxidant vitamins, which makes it a recommended food against diabetes, heart disease, hypertension or cancer.

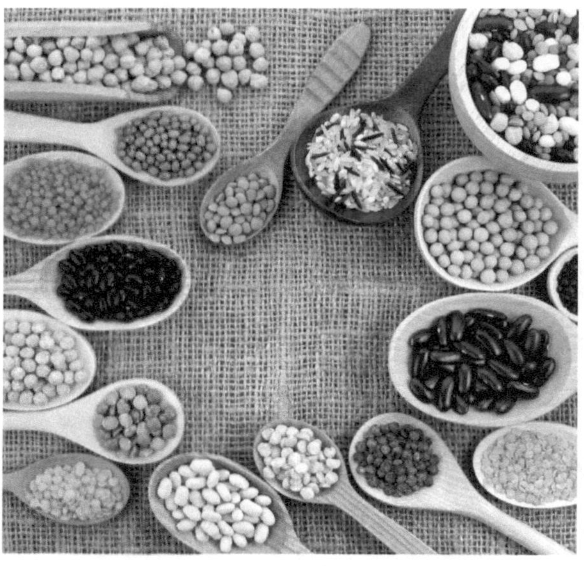

They have a lot of calories but they help in weight loss, not letting you feel hungry easily.

I eat them often, in small servings and without much olive oil to avoid adding even more calories.

Along with legumes I have a slice of whole wheat bread, a salad — broccoli, cauliflower, wild chicories (in all cases with olive oil and lemon), but most often tomatoes (with olive oil, oregano, thyme and onion) — and a glass of wine.

## Tuesday

In Tuesday I enjoy a bream, my favorite fish, usually with wild chicories, or with a salad of potatoes, zucchinis, tomatoes, oregano, thyme, onion, or any other simple salad, of course with olive oil.

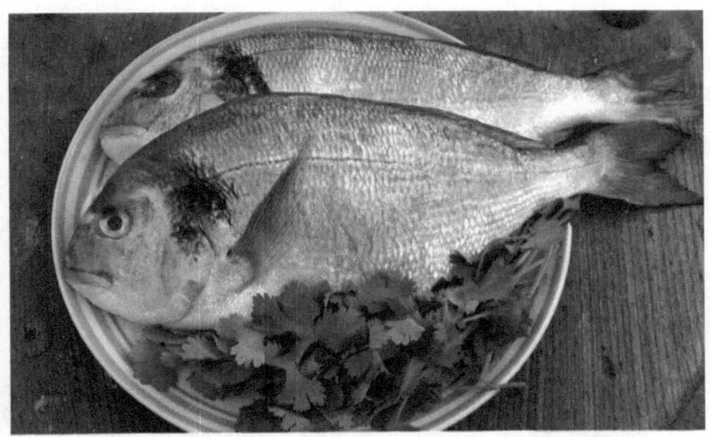

I cook my bream in the oven's grill, I n e v e r fry it, n e v e r let it be cooked in its fat or in anything else, I never add garlic or whatever.

The best way to enjoy the subtle taste of a bream is to make it in the grill, 10–15 minutes each side, then serve as it is, or adding just a tablespoon of olive oil and some lemon drops.

I like wine with anything, but I wouldn't say no to a nice beer with my bream. A slice of fresh whole wheat bread is also necessary!

## Wednesday

The day of the eggs! I prefer two fried eggs, but when I need to avoid some calories, I make them an omelet and use less oil.

As always, a salad is there, tomatoes with olive oil, etc., and a slice or two of whole wheat bread. Wine of course, or beer.

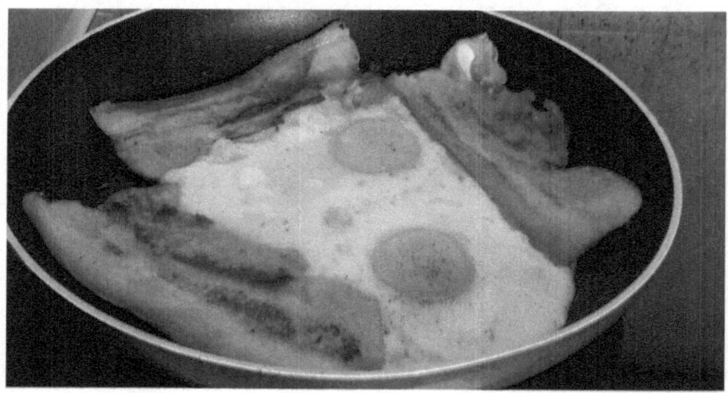

Now sometimes I make this exception, to fry also bacon, a rather useless but tasty kind of a "meat", in which case I fry my eggs in bacon's fat without adding oil.

Of course on Wednesdays I never have eggs as a breakfast!

## Friday

Tuna Day! One of my favorite meals! Of course I use tuna canned in w a t e r, which I cook without oil at all, just some chopped tomatoes, onion, basil, salt, pepper, a shot of white wine, and a small spoon of honey.

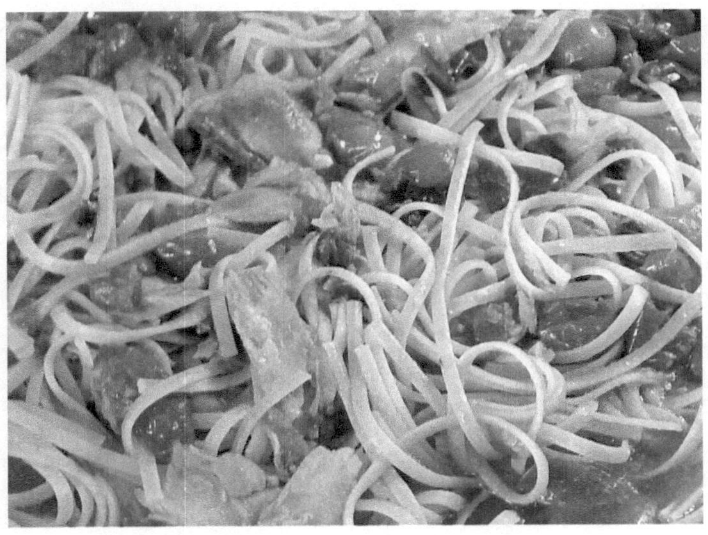

I boil whole wheat spaghetti separately, and I serve them with the tuna sauce at the top and Regato light cheese. A very simple and delicious recipe that needs just 15 minutes! Sometimes I use shrimps instead of tuna.

I don't like a salad with this dish, just wine or beer.


## Saturday


A free day; I cook whatever I miss most, even not–so–healthy food, usually my home made pizza!

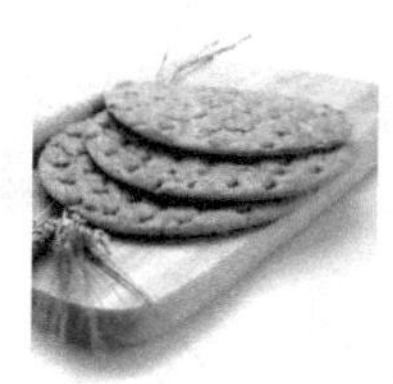

I prepare my personal pizza using whole wheat "pita", an available in stores rather thick dough that is used in the Greek "souvlaki", a street food usually containing slices of pork and tomatoes. I use this pie for my pizza and I add a lot of fresh tomatoes (thin slices), mushrooms, perhaps some bacon, and also red, orange and yellow peppers (never green, because their taste is so sharp, it covers everything!), no oil at all, Mozzarella and Gouda cheese, salt, pepper and basil.

Contrary to the pizza that we order, in this one each of the main ingredients occupies a whole level: there is no piece of tomato *beside* a mushroom, for instance. There is a whole level of tomatoes, then a whole level of mushrooms, etc. Cheese is above everything, unless I add also a few pieces of bacon.

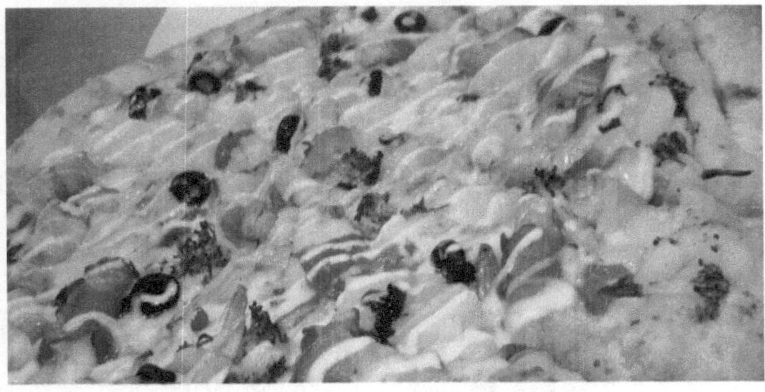

In the end my pizza seems like a mountain, but being baked it shrinks. In the (all over in maximum temperature preheated) oven it needs just 10 minutes and it's ready! It equals in size about two and a half pieces of a pizza you can order, but it's a lot healthier. Wine, Coke (with Stevia instead of sugar), or a beer are equally welcome in this table.

## Sunday

The day of red meat, poultry, or a delicious rabbit...

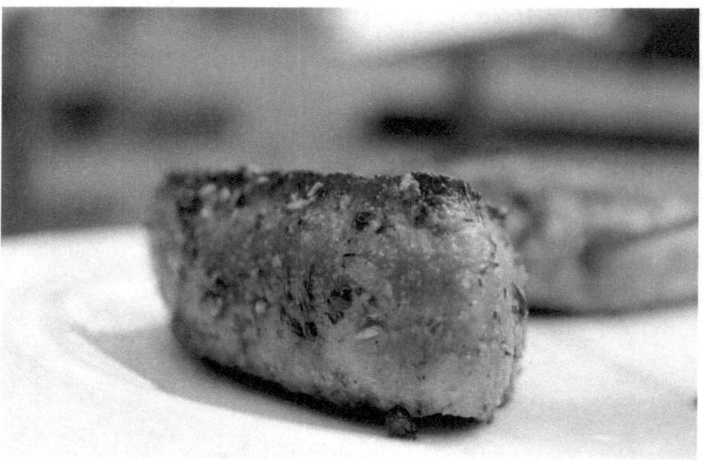

For red meat I prefer a steak cooked without oil, sometimes a low–fat part of pork, or calf meat with tomato sauce without much oil, and in all cases whole wheat pasta, or rice.

Chicken or turkey can be made in the exact same ways. I only eat rabbit with red sauce containing or not whole onions.

A tomato salad is great with all of these dishes, along with wine or beer, but of course any salad is fine, without sauces and the like, just olive oil and lemon, if you prefer chicories, or broccoli, or cauliflower; olive oil and oregano, thyme and onion, if your prefer a salad of tomatoes, zucchini, potatoes, etc.

## Making up your own schedule

You don't need to imitate each and every detail I give here, but let everything inspire you in your own efforts and pleasures, always following the general rules — moderate use of olive oil, eating legumes, avoiding anything fried and anything made of white flour, eating only whole wheat bread and pasta, drinking a lot of water, drinking wine, etc.

*The overall sense should be that of moderation, quality, health, balance, variety.*

Keep this idea of having a schedule, rotating as many recipes as you like but in some order, and keeping a measure in all of your meals — never be *glutted like beasts.*

A schedule helps to judge your choices and arrive soon at a final form that works best for you.

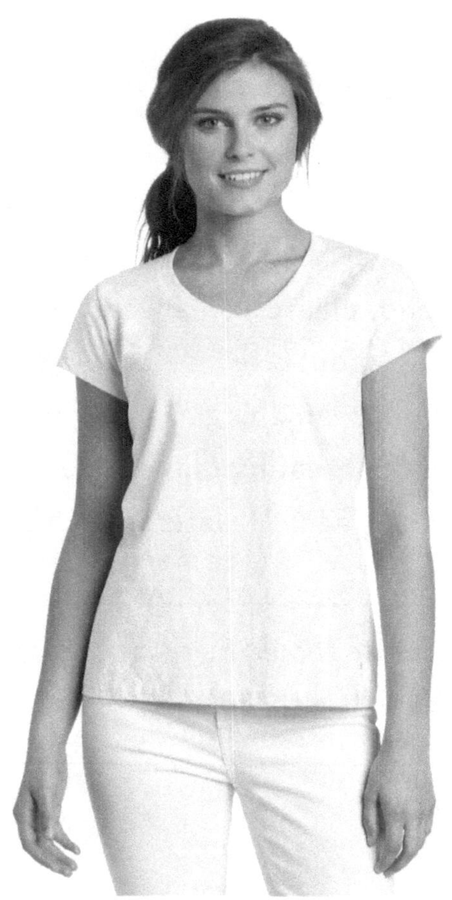

# Recipes you want to try

I'm sharing these recipes first of all because I like them, but also because they support my own efforts to avoid unnecessary weight. Nothing strange, most of them belonging to the Mediterranean diet, which I modified to become lower in calories while remaining equally healthy and tasty.

## *Bean soup*

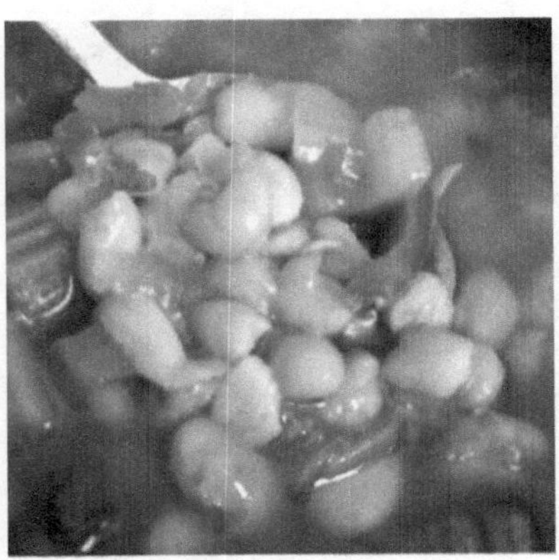

### Ingredients (5 servings)

*500 g dry white beans*
*3 medium onions*

*1 bunch of celery*
*6 medium carrots*
*80 ml extra virgin olive oil*
*100 g chopped tomatoes*
*Salt*
*Pepper*

### Directions

The night before we cook the beans, we let them in a bowl of water covering them.

In the morning we put them in a pot, adding as much water as needed to cover them fully. When boil begins we lower the fire and let them simmer for about 50 minutes. Then we need to taste and see if they are ready because that depends on the quality of our beans. If they are still hard, we let them simmer even more; after a while we taste again.

When they are ready, we add the vegetables in small pieces, along with 3 spoons of olive oil and chopped tomatoes. We continue simmering until the soup starts to thicken.

We add some salt, pepper, and the remaining olive oil, and we are ready to serve, accompanying with salted fish, pickled vegetables, and olives. Whole wheat bread and good red wine are necessary!

## Chickpea soup

### Ingredients (5 servings)

*500 g chickpeas*
*80 ml extra virgin olive oil*
*1 large onion grated*
*5 strands of dill, finely chopped*
*Juice of 2 lemons*
*Salt*
*Pepper*

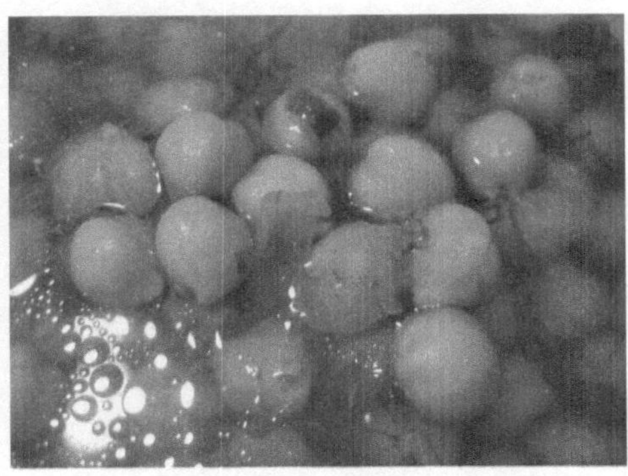

### Directions

The night before we cook them, we let the chickpeas in a bowl of water that covers them completely.

In the morning we put them in a pot, we cover them with water and we let them boil. For 5–10 minutes we skim them; when they are clean we add the onion, oil, and dill, and we lower the heat letting them simmer for about one and a half hours.

This depends on the quality of our chickpeas; you need to taste once in a while to avoid making them too soft or leaving them too hard.

When they are ready we increase the fire, we add salt and the lemon juice, and let them have 2–3 boils. Finally we add pepper, and that's it!

Serve with salted fish, olives, and any salad you like, whole wheat bread, and wine or beer.

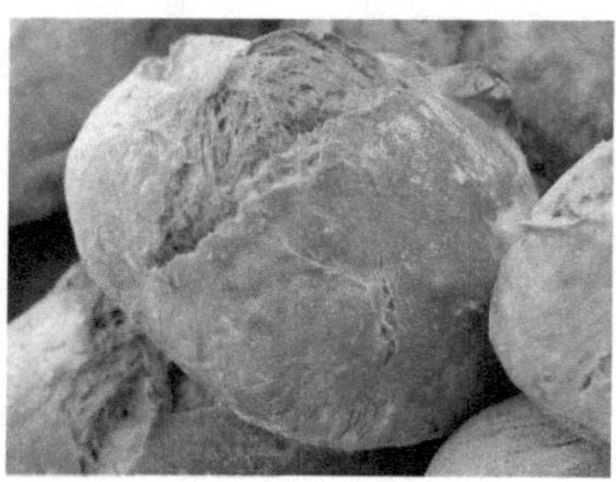

# Lima (giant) beans in the oven

Ingredients (for 6 servings)

500 g lima beans
70 g extra virgin olive oil
1 dry onion
2 fresh onions
2 cloves of garlic
2 bay leaves
1 t. honey
500 ml chopped tomatoes
50 g white wine
Zest from 1 lemon
1 t. rosemary
300 g water
Salt
Pepper

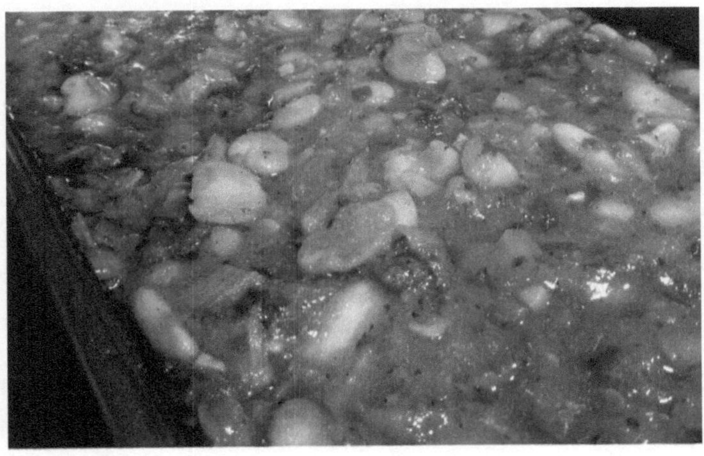

### Directions

We put the beans in a bowl of salted water for the night. In the morning we strain them and we pour water to remove any salt left.

We put them in a saucepan, add water, and transfer them to the fire letting them simmer for 1 hour. Then we strain them and put them aside.

In the same saucepan we mix the olive oil with the onion, celery, pepper, chopped garlic, the bay leaves, honey, and tomatoes. We let them boil for a few minutes and we pour white wine. When alcohol is evaporated we mix water, lemon zest, rosemary, pepper, salt, and the beans.

We preheat the oven to 180° C (air).

We transfer the beans to a baking pan (about 20x40 cm) and we add the fresh onions chopped. We cover with an aluminum foil and bake for about 1 hour, but tasting once in a while to see if they have become soft enough. Then we uncover the pan and continue cooking for about 10 minutes to let more water evaporate.

We serve with any salad we like, whole wheat bread, and wine or beer.

## Lentil soup

Ingredients (5 servings)

300 g lentils
30 g extra virgin olive oil
500 ml chopped tomatoes
1 large onion
3 cloves of garlic
1 TB. fresh ginger
3 carrots cleaned
1 liter of water
Salt
Pepper

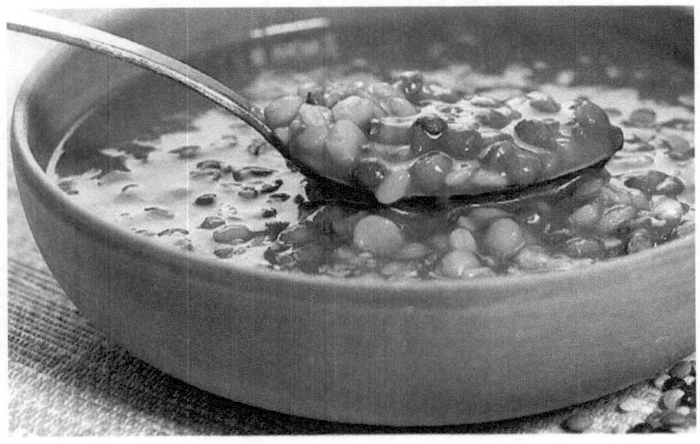

### Directions

Grate the ginger, onion and garlic and put them in a saucepan. Cut the carrots into thin slices, and add them. Finally, add the lentils, water, tomatoes, salt and pepper. Let them simmer for 30 minutes or until lentils soften.

Serve with any salad you like, salted fish, whole wheat bread, and wine or beer.

# Green beans with beef

### Ingredients (5 servings)

*450 g green beans*
*1 kg low-fat beef*
*4 TB. olive oil*
*2 carrots*
*50 g white wine*
*1 liter of water*
*1 TB. parsley*
*1 TB. anise*
*1 TB. mint*
*1 dry onion*
*1 fresh onion*
*1 clove of garlic*

*Juice and zest of 2 lemons*
*Salt*
*Pepper*

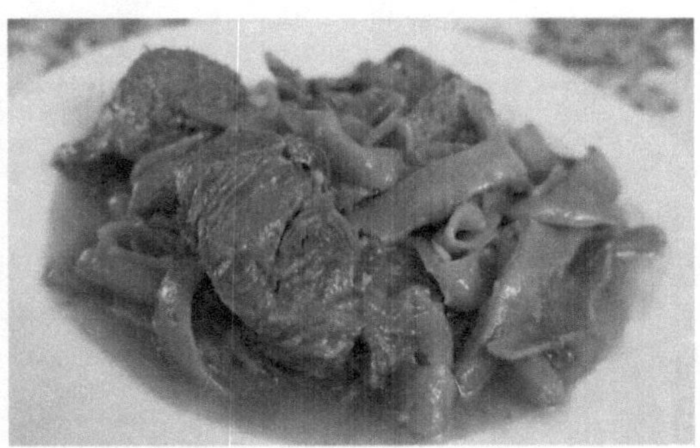

Directions

Cut the beef into (not too small) pieces and put it in a saucepan with salt and pepper. Cut the carrots, crumble the onion and the garlic. Add them along with the wine and the water. Simmer for about an hour and a half. Then add the beans.

Fold the leaves of parsley, dill and mint and put them in a bowl. Cut the green part of the fresh onion into small slices and put them in the bowl. Add lemon zest and mix.

Put the herbs in the sauce with lemon juice. Simmer for 10 minutes. Just make sure that beans won't become too soft; they should be *al dente!*

No need for salad of course; serve with whole wheat bread, and wine or beer.

# Split peas (fava)

Ingredients  (5 servings)

*250 g split peas*
*1 dry onion, whole*
*4 dry onions cut into fine frames*
*10 TB olive oil*
*Juice of two lemons*
*Salt and pepper*

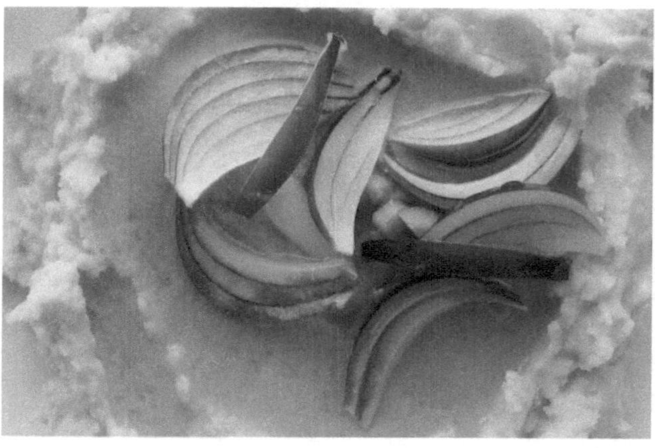

## Directions

We put the split peas in a moderate pot with 1 liter of water. Once it boils, we lower the fire and for the first 10 minutes scrape it thoroughly.

Then we add the whole onion, and we let the peas simmer, stirring occasionally, for 40 minutes or until they are softened, having absorbed all water.

When it is ready, we pour salt, pepper, two tablespoons of oil and the lemon juice. We stir well until it becomes puree.

For each serving we add a lot of chopped onion covering its surface along with 2 tablespoons of olive oil.

We can enjoy it with octopus or salted fish, and of course with whole wheat bread, and wine.

## *Roast beef with pasta*

### Ingredients (6 servings)

*1 kg of a calf; any low-fat part is fine*

*4 cloves of garlic*
*5 TB. olive oil*
*1 large dry onion (very well chopped)*
*1 carrot*
*1 bunch of celery*
*500 ml chopped tomatoes*
*A cup of white wine*
*1 bay leaf*
*Allspice (pimento)*
*Clove*
*Salt*
*Pepper*
*1 pack (500 g) of thick pasta*
*Regato light, chopped*

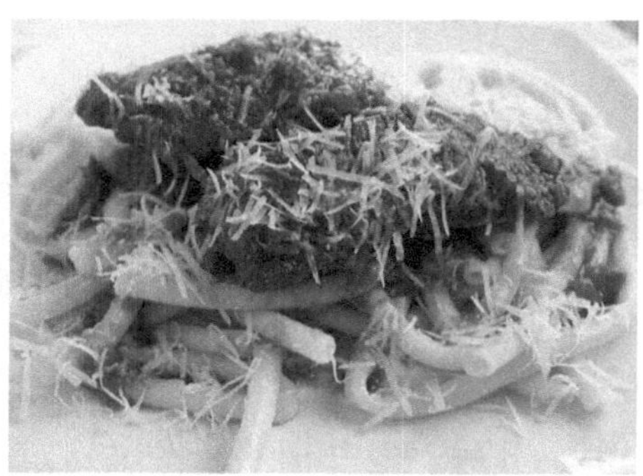

## Directions

We salt the meat, then we chop garlic in thick pieces to bury them in various places into the meat.

We roast very well all around the meat in a pot with a tablespoon of olive oil. We add the wine and we let it evaporate.

Then we add the vegetables, the rest of the olive oil, the tomatoes, a little water and we let the meat simmer until it becomes soft and the sauce thickens.

Then we cut it into large pieces and we let it simmer for 5 minutes more. We add spices, salt and pepper, and we serve with thick pasta or whole wheat linguini and Regato light.

Any salad is fine, and of course beer or wine.

## A hunter's rabbit

Ingredients (5 servings)

*1 big rabbit in portions*
*1 glass of vinegar*
*10 large cloves of garlic chopped*
*100 ml olive oil*
*800 ml chopped tomatoes*
*2-3 bay leaves*

*Salt and pepper*
*1 lemon juice*

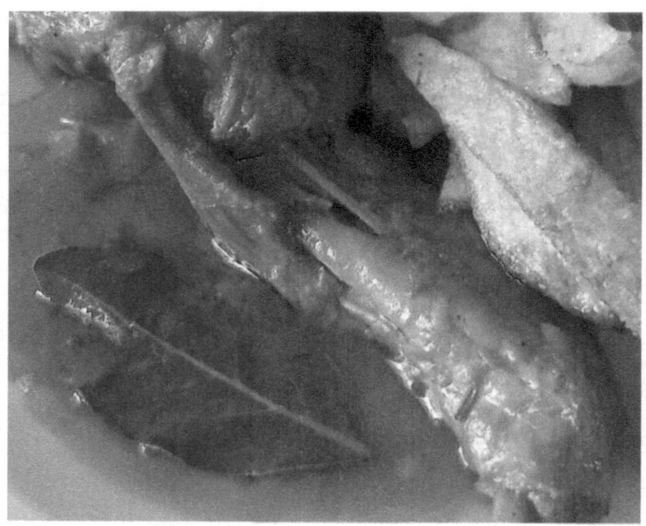

### Directions

We put the rabbit in a deep bowl with the vinegar and keep it in the refrigerator for the night. In the morning we rinse it with water and wipe it well with kitchen towels.

In a frying pan we add the rabbit with a tablespoon of olive oil and we rotate it a few times until it turns brown.

In a large pot we pour the olive oil, the chopped garlic cloves, the tomatoes, bay leaves, salt and pepper and let them boil. Then we add the rabbit pieces and, if necessary, some water.

We have to let the food simmer for 2–3 hours, until it is left with a thick juice. Finally we pour the lemon juice and leave the fire on for half an hour.

We serve with fried potatoes, or if we prefer a healthier option, with rice or whole wheat spaghetti.

Any salad is fine, and wine or beer.

## Bream in grill

So easy, you don't need more details than what I said above, in the "Tuesday" part of my weekly schedule.

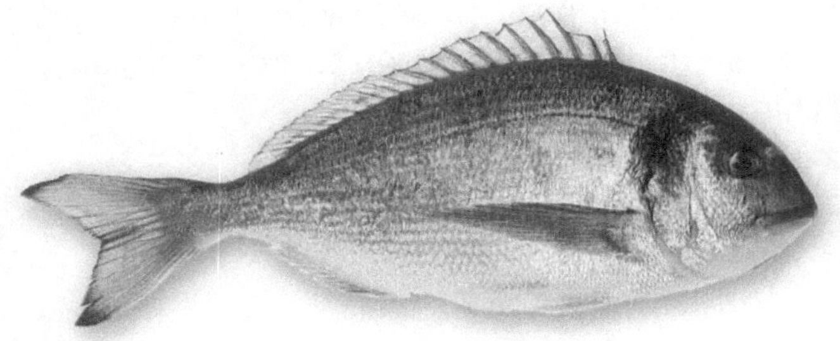

# Tuna with pasta

One of my favorite dishes, and it's made in 15 minutes. Just see an overview (more than enough) above, in the "Friday" part.

# Home made pizza

Well, not all of it is home made, since I buy the base, but a base made of a thick whole–wheat pastry. You can read the rest at the "Saturday" part of my schedule.

# Minced meat with pasta

Ingredients (5 servings)

*1 kg of calf minced (any low-fat part is fine; you can also use minced chicken or turkey and you won't enjoy this recipe less!)*
*2 onions chopped*
*2 cloves of garlic chopped*
*A shot of cognac*

*Juice of one orange*
*500 ml chopped tomatoes*
*2 bay leaves*
*1 t. pimento powder*
*1/3 t. cinnamon*
*1 t. nutmeg*
*1 bunch of parsley*
*1 t. honey*
*Salt*
*Pepper*
*1 pack (500 g) whole wheat spaghetti*
*Regato cheese light grated*

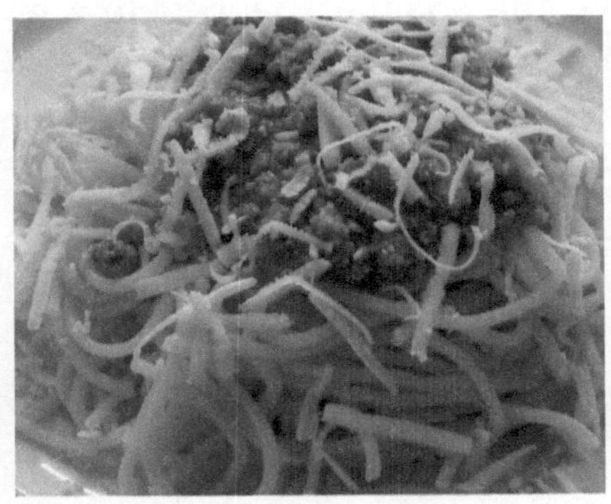

## Directions

Heat a saucepan without olive oil or anything and roast the mince for about 7 minutes to brown it, without stirring a lot, to avoid boiling it in its juice.

Add the chopped onion and garlic, the cognac and orange juice, tomatoes, and the bay leaves. Add a little water and let it simmer for about half an hour.

Finally, add salt and pepper, the spices, parsley and honey. Simmer for about 10 minutes more, until the sauce is thick enough. Remove the bay leaves and parsley bunch.

Serve it above the spaghetti and below grated cheese.

Wine or beer is fine, and any salad you may like. I prefer to enjoy it without a salad, though.

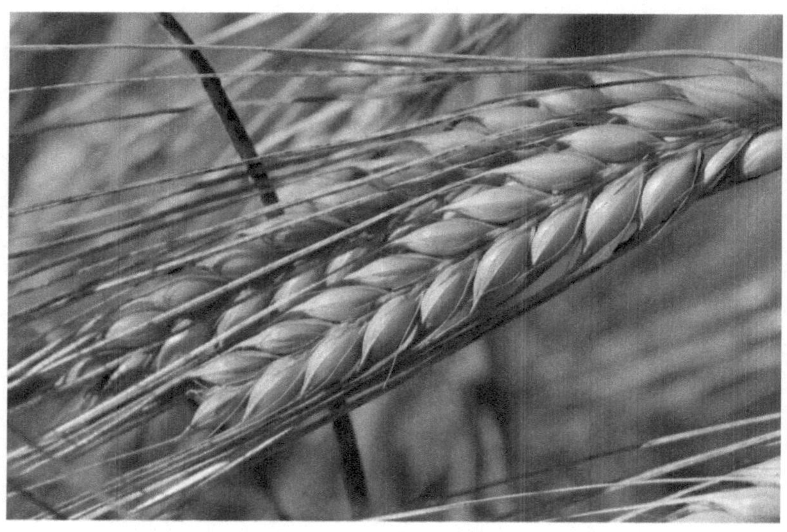

# Some important food calories

The purpose of the following list is not to help you add amounts of calories to calculate meticulously some ideal combinations for daily meals. It would be a burdensome and tedious task you don't even need. Having to calculate calories for the rest of your life to prepare your meals! It's exhausting, it's just not feasible, and most probably you'll find yourself sooner or later gaining the weight you lost, and you'll have to fight also with despair. It helps though to form a rough idea of what foods are high or low in calories, just to be cautious. Since you need to eat any healthy food, having an idea about calories will help you exercise your moderation.

Eating only when you are really hungry, sleeping well, drinking a lot of water, and aiming at losing your appetite rather than being satiated, combined with the avoidance of junk food and the moderate use of high–calorie healthy foods, will be cultivating *easy, spontaneous and effective* dietary habits, able to help you lose as much weight as you need, especially if you devote also some time in light exercise, and, more than that, will make you able to keep your normal weight and avoid getting fat in the future, since they change your whole food attitude.

Red Meat

| | | |
|---|---|---|
| Beef shoulder, without fat | 85 g | 183 |
| Beef steak without fat | 85 g | 174 |
| Beef, chest, cooked | 85 g | 189 |
| Beef, minced and cooked | 85 g | 245 |
| Kebab | 85 g | 226 |
| Lamb rib, grilled with fat | 85 g | 307 |
| Lamb rib, grilled without fat | 85 g | 200 |
| Lamb shoulder, cooked with fat | 63 g | 220 |
| Lamb shoulder, cooked without fat | 48 g | 135 |
| Lamb thigh, roasted with fat | 85 g | 205 |
| Lamb thigh, roasted without fat | 73 g | 140 |
| Pork shoulder, lean and fat, roast | 28 g | 75 |
| Pork, sausage, large, grilled, each | | 160 |
| Pork, shoulder, lean, roast only | 28 g | 58 |

Poultry

| | | |
|---|---|---|
| Chicken leg (hip), without skin, grilled | 85 g | 167 |
| Chicken leg (hip), with skin, grilled | 85 g | 223 |
| Chicken breast, without skin, grilled | Half a breast | 142 |

| | | |
|---|---|---|
| Chicken breast, with skin, grilled | Half a breast | 193 |
| Chicken breast, without skin, fried | Half a breast | 161 |
| Chicken wings, with skin, grilled | 1 wing "35.5 g" | 99 |
| Chicken pieces, vacuum, fried | 6 pieces "104 g" | 290 |
| Chicken gizzards, fried | 85 g | 238 |
| Chicken livers, cooked | 85 g | 135 |
| Duck meat, without skin, roasted | 85 g | 173 |
| Turkey Red dark meat, without skin | 85 g | 161 |
| Turkey Red dark meat, with skin | 85 g | 190 |
| Turkey Red light meat, meat without skin | 85 g | 135 |
| Turkey Red light meat, meat with skin | 85 g | 169 |

## Fish & Shellfish

| | | |
|---|---|---|
| Anchovies, canned in oil | 21 g | 42 |
| Caviar, black or red | 1 tablespoon | 40 |
| Crab, canned | 85 g | 84 |
| Fish fried with rusk | 3 pieces, 85 g | 228 |
| Grilled Fish | 85 g | 136 |
| Oyster, uncooked | 28 g | 23 |
| Oysters, fried | 28 g | 46 |
| Oysters, fried with rusk | 85 g | 84 |
| Sardines, canned in oil | 28 g | 58 |
| Shrimp fried with rusk | 85 g | 206 |
| Shrimp, cooked | 85 g | 83 |
| Smoked salmon | 85 g | 99 |
| Tuna, canned in oil | 85 g | 169 |

| | | |
|---|---|---|
| Tuna, canned in water | 85 g | 104 |

## Milk & Cheese

| | | |
|---|---|---|
| Full-fat milk | 1 cup | 150 |
| Low fat milk (1%) | 1 cup | 102 |
| Cow's milk | 1 cup | 157 |
| Goat milk | 1 cup | 264 |
| Full cream milk powder | Half a cup | 635 |
| Skim milk powder | Half a cup | 435 |
| Full-fat chocolate milk | 1 cup | 208 |
| Strawberry Milk | 1 cup | 244 |
| Cheddar cheese slices | Slice, 28 g | 114 |
| Feta cheese | 28 g | 75 |
| Gouda cheese | 28 g | 101 |
| Mozzarella cheese | 28 g | 80 |
| Kraft Cheese "cups" | 28 g | 80 |
| Edam cheese | 28 g | 98 |
| Blue cheese | 28 g | 104 |
| Parmesan cheese | 28 g | 130 |
| Cottage cheese | 100 g | 99 |
| Cream focused | 1 spoon | 52 |
| Cream Medium | 1 spoon | 37 |

### Ice Cream

| | | |
|---|---|---|
| Vanilla | 1 ball | 240 |
| Cocoa | 1 ball | 280 |
| Strawberries | 1 ball | 220 |

## Drinks, Juices

| | | |
|---|---|---|
| Apple juice | Half a cup | 60 |
| Apricot juice, canned | Half a cup | 72 |
| Grape juice, canned | Half a cup | 78 |
| Lemon juice canned | Spoon to eat | 3 |
| Fresh orange juice | Half a cup | 59 |
| Canned orange juice | Half a cup | 52 |
| Grapefruit juice, canned local | Half a cup | 58 |
| Grapefruit juice, unsweetened | Half a cup | 47 |
| Canned peach juice | Half a cup | 67 |
| Canned pear juice | Half a cup | 75 |
| Canned pineapple juice | Half a cup | 70 |
| Canned tomato juice | Half a cup | 21 |
| Mango juice | One cup | 110 |

| | | |
|---|---|---|
| Nescafe without sugar | Teaspoon | 5 |
| Instant coffee without caffeine | Teaspoon | 5 |
| Tea without sugar | One cup | 1 |
| American coffee | One cup | 5 |

| | | |
|---|---|---|
| Pepsi-Cola | 240 ml cup | 100 |
| Diet Pepsi-Cola | 240 ml cup | 0.00 |
| Seven Up | 240 ml cup | 90 |
| Sprite | 240 ml cup | 96 |
| Fanta | 240 ml cup | 119 |
| Coca-Cola | 240 ml cup | 97 |

| | | |
|---|---|---|
| Diet Coca-Cola | 240 ml cup | 1.00 |
| Cream soda | 240 ml cup | 126 |
| Drink grape gas | 240 ml cup | 107 |

## Eggs

| | | |
|---|---|---|
| Egg whites, (fresh or iced) | One, big | 17 |
| Fresh egg yolk | One, big | 59 |
| Full cook boiled eggs | One, big | 79 |
| Fried eggs | One, big | 91 |
| Omelet | One, big | 92 |
| Omelet with cheese and vegetables | 113 g | 252 |
| Duck eggs | One, big | 130 |
| Goose eggs | One, big | 267 |
| Turkey eggs | One, big | 135 |
| Quail eggs | One, big | 14 |

## Nuts & Legumes

| | | |
|---|---|---|
| Nuts | Half a cup, 60 g | 380 |
| Almonds, dry | Quarter a cup | 209 |
| Cashew, roasted, dry | 28 g | 160 |
| Cashew, roasted, oily | 28 g | 165 |
| Nuts, roasted, dry | 28 g | 170 |
| Hazelnut, roasted, oily | 28 g | 176 |
| Lentils, whole, green | Half a cup | 215 |
| Lentils, cooked | One cup | 210 |

| | | |
|---|---|---|
| Beans, boiled | One cup | 187 |
| Dry beans | One cup | 349 |
| Chickpeas, boiled | Half a cup | 269 |
| Flour | One cup | 339 |
| Lentil | Half a cup | 192 |
| Nuts mixed with roasted and dry peanuts | 28 g | 170 |
| Mixed nuts roasted in oil | 28 g | 175 |
| Sunflower seeds, roasted and dry | 28 g | 170 |
| Sunflower seed, roasted in oil | 28 g | 175 |
| Pistachios, dry and roasted | Half a cup | 357 |
| Peanuts, dry and roasted | 28 g | 165 |
| Peanuts, roasted in oil | 28 g | 170 |
| Peanut butter | Spoon 16 g | 95 |
| Roasted chestnut | 28 g | 44 |
| Coconut | 28 g | 100 |
| Grated coconut | 28 g | 59 |
| Roasted pumpkin seeds | 28 g | 127 |
| Dried watermelon seeds | 28 g | 158 |
| Circuit pills | 28 g | 102.2 |
| Sesame | 28 g | 174.16 |
| Pine | 28 g | 172.7 |

Fresh Fruits

| | | |
|---|---|---|
| Apples | Medium, 140 g | 81 |
| Apricot | Medium, 30 g | 17 |
| Banana | Medium, 100 g | 105 |

| | | |
|---|---|---|
| Fig | One, 40 g | 37 |
| Grapefruit | Half | 38 |
| Cherries | 10 beads | 49 |
| Avocado | Half | 162 |
| Grapes | Half a cup | 53 |
| Guava | One, 85 g | 45 |
| Kiwi | One, 76 g | 46 |
| Mango | Half, 85 g | 68 |
| Orange | One, 110 g | 62 |
| Papaya | Medium | 117 |
| Peach | One, 85 g | 37 |
| Pear | Medium, 170 g | 98 |
| Pineapple | Slice, 82 g | 42 |
| Plum | One, 60 g | 36 |
| Pomegranate | Medium, 150 g | 110 |
| Nectarine | Medium, 142 g | 67 |
| Watermelon | Piece, 100 g | 26 |
| Melon | Piece, 100 g | 33 |
| Strawberries | Half a cup | 23 |
| Tangerine | One, 85 g | 37 |
| Blueberry | One cup | 122 |
| Loquat | 100 g | 49 |
| Plum | 100 g | 52 |
| Lemon | One, 60 g | 17 |
| Sweet Lemon | Fruit size | 53 |
| Black berry | One cup | 117 |
| Quince | Medium | 60 |
| Tamarind | Half a cup | 82 |

## Canned Fruits

| | | |
|---|---|---|
| Canned apricots (with sugar syrup) | Half a cup | 111 |
| Fruit salad (with sugar syrup) | Half a cup | 94 |
| Canned cherry (with thick sugar syrup) | Half a cup | 107 |
| Canned peaches (with sugar syrup) | Half a cup | 95 |
| Canned pear with (with sugar syrup) | Half a cup | 94 |
| Canned pineapple (with sugar syrup) | Half a cup | 100 |

## Dried Fruits

| | | |
|---|---|---|
| Dried dates | One | 26 |
| Dried figs | 100 g | 288 |
| Raisins | Half a cup | 109 |
| Dried plum | Half a cup | 113 |
| Dried Apricots | Half a cup | 169 |

## Spices

| | | |
|---|---|---|
| Cardamon | 1 teaspoon | 7 |
| Dried hot red pepper | 3 teaspoons | 13 |
| Cinnamon | 1 teaspoon | 7 |
| Cloves | 1 teaspoon | 6 |
| Latency | 1 teaspoon | 6 |
| Ginger "powder" | 1 teaspoon | 1 |

| | | |
|---|---|---|
| Ginger root | One, medium | 20 |
| Nutmeg "powder" | 1 teaspoon | 9 |
| Black pepper | 1 teaspoon | 8 |

## Vegetables

| | | |
|---|---|---|
| Carrot | Medium, 60 g | 31 |
| Carrot, cooked | Half a cup | 35 |
| Cauliflower, cooked | Half a cup | 15 |
| Cauliflower, uncooked | Half a cup | 12 |
| Cucumbers, chopped | Half a cup | 7 |
| Fried eggplant | Half a cup | 100 |
| Eggplant, cooked | Half a cup | 13 |
| Green beans, cooked | Half a cup | 20 |
| Green beans, canned | Half a cup | 25 |
| Cabbage, cooked | Half a cup | 16 |
| Cabbage, uncooked | Half a cup | 8 |
| Celery | Half a cup | 10 |
| Corn | One, medium | 77 |
| Mushrooms, fresh | Half a cup | 9 |
| Mushroom, canned | Half a cup | 19 |
| Lettuce | Half a cup | 4 |
| Mixed vegetables | Half a cup | 54 |
| Okra, cooked and chopped | Half a cup | 25 |
| Fresh onions, chopped | Half a cup | 27 |
| Green onions, chopped | Half a cup | 16 |
| Green peas, cooked | Half a cup | 67 |
| Peppers, chopped | Half a cup | 12 |

| | | |
|---|---|---|
| Hot pepper | One, 30 g | 18 |
| Baked potato, with the peel | 195 g | 220 |
| Baked potato, without the peel | 195 g | 162 |
| Fried potato | 10 pieces, 42 g | 158 |
| Watercress | Half a cup | 2 |
| Squash | Half a cup | 41 |
| Chopped spinach | Half a cup | 6 |
| Zucchini, chopped and cooked | Half a cup | 18 |
| Sweet potatoes, mashed | Half a cup | 111 |
| Red tomatoes | One, medium | 26 |
| Green beans | One cup | 73 |
| Beet | One cup | 46 |
| Cabbage | One cup | 73 |
| Leek | 1 Spoon, minced | 1 |
| Coriander | 1 package | 97 |
| Fenugreek, leaves | 1 package | 25 |
| Garlic | 5 pieces of garlic peeled | 7 |
| Grape leaves | 1 cup | 146 |
| Mint | Package, medium | 84 |
| Black olives | 10 grains, medium | 95 |
| Green olives | 10 grains, medium | 66 |
| Olive oil | 1 TB | 155 |
| Parsley | 1 cup, minced | 34 |
| Parsley | Package, medium | 25 |
| Spinach | 1 Cup, chopped | 14 |
| Zucchini | One, medium | 40 |

| | | |
|---|---|---|
| Basil | 100 g | 50 |
| Boil | 100 g | 32 |
| Legume | 100 g | 32 |
| Sugar-cane | 100 g | 82 |

Grains

| | | |
|---|---|---|
| Whole wheat bread | One, 50 g | 130 |
| Pasta with sauce | Small, 130 g | 190 |
| Corn flakes | Cup, 25 g | 95 |
| French bread | Quarter of a loaf, 115 g | 333 |
| Plain biscuits | 4 pieces, 55 g | 178 |
| White rice, cooked (long grain) | Half a cup | 131 |
| Brown toast | A slice | 61 |
| Plain white toast | A slice | 64 |
| Spaghetti | Half a cup | 99 |
| Spaghetti with minced meat and tomato | Half a cup | 110 |
| Lasagna with meat sauce | Half a cup | 154 |
| Barley | One cup | 672 |
| Pasta | One cup | 344 |
| Rice, uncooked | One cup | 675 |
| Rice powder | One cup | 354 |
| Wheat | One cup | 485 |

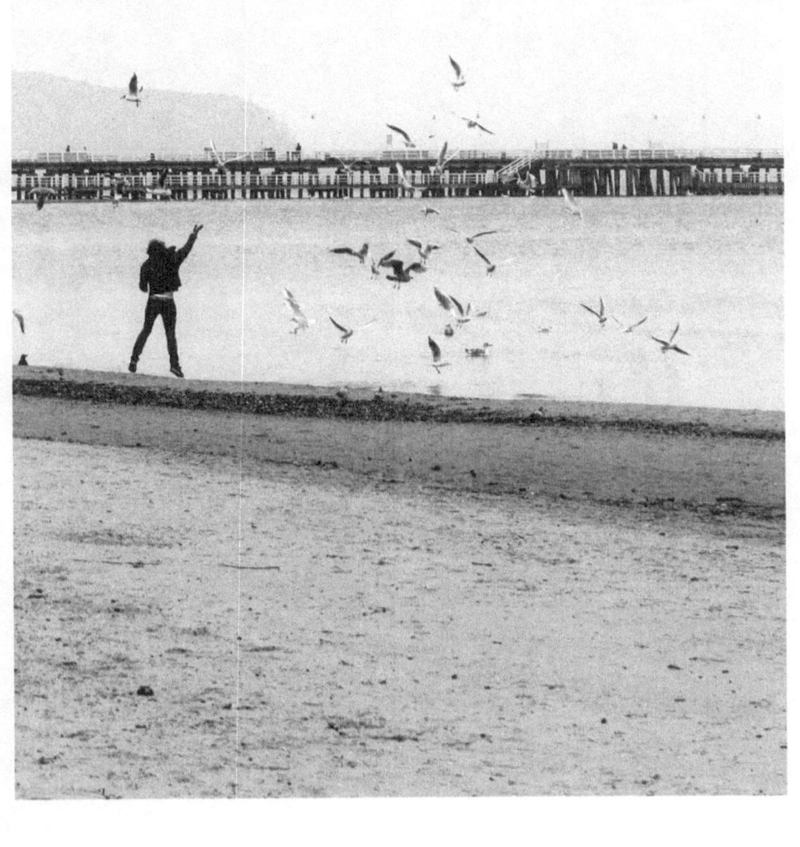

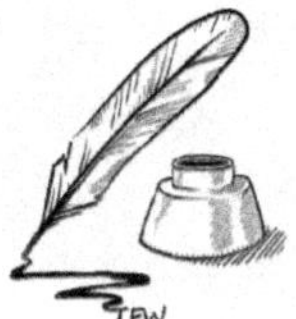

www.ingramcontent.com/pod-product-compliance
Lightning Source LLC
Chambersburg PA
CBHW031418250726
48656CB00002B/720